# HYPERTHYROIDISM DIET PLAN COOK BOOK

## A Complete Diet Plan with Specific Recipes for People With Hyperthyroidism.

**REX LEWIS**

# Table of Contents

# Introduction

Hyperthyroidism Is A State When The Thyroid Gland Is Overly Active, Resulting In An Excessive Release Of Thyroid Hormones. These Hormones Are Essential For Controlling Many Body Activities, Such As Metabolism. Treating Hyperthyroidism Typically Requires A Mix Of Medication Intervention And Lifestyle Modifications, Such As Changes In Nutrition.

Diet Cannot Cure Hyperthyroidism, But It Can Help Reduce Symptoms And Promote General Well-Being. The Main Objectives Of A Hyperthyroidism Diet Are To Supply Essential Nutrients, Boost Energy Levels, And Maybe Assist

In Controlling Weight Changes Linked To The Illness.

**Here are some broad recommendations for a diet suitable for those with hyperthyroidism:**

**1. Ensure A Balanced Intake Of Nutrients.**

• Ensure A Diet That Includes A Variety Of Carbohydrates, Proteins, And Fats To Maintain Equilibrium.

• Incorporate A Diverse Range Of Fruits, Vegetables, Whole Grains, Lean Meats, And Healthy Fats Into Your Meals.

## 2.  Avoid  Excessive  Use  Of Stimulants.

• Avoid Or Minimize Stimulants Like Caffeine And Nicotine, As They Can Worsen Symptoms Such As Anxiety And Insomnia.

## 3. Avoid Foods High In Iodine.

• Excessive Iodine Intake Might Exacerbate Hyperthyroidism In Some Situations. Restrict Intake Of Iodine-Rich Foods Such As Seaweed, Iodized Salt, And Specific Seafood.

## 4. Calcium and Vitamin D:

• Hyperthyroidism Can Impact Bone Health. Consume Sufficient Calcium And Vitamin D From Dairy Products,

Leafy Greens, Fortified Foods, Or Supplements If Needed.

**5. Regular, Frequent Meals:**

• Eating Smaller, More Frequent Meals Can Aid In Managing Weight Changes Linked To Hyperthyroidism.

**6. Moisture:** Stay Well-Hydrated By Drinking Enough Water. Dehydration Can Lead To Weariness And Other Symptoms.

**7. Work Together With A Healthcare Professional:**

• Collaborate With Your Healthcare Team, Including A Licensed Dietitian Or Nutritionist, To Customize Your Diet According To Your Individual

Requirements And Track Your Nutritional Well-Being.

It Is Important To Recognize That Individual Reactions To Dietary Modifications Might Differ, And What Is Effective For One People May Not Be Effective For Another. Prior To Making Substantial Alterations To Your Diet, It Is Advisable To Seek Guidance From Your Healthcare Professional, Particularly If You Have A Medical Condition Such As Hyperthyroidism. They Can Offer Tailored Guidance According To Your Individual Health Requirements And Factors To Consider.

# CHAPTER ONE
## Overview of Hyperthyroidism

Hyperthyroidism Is A Disorder When The Thyroid Gland Is Overly Active, Resulting In An Excessive Production Of Thyroid Hormones. The Thyroid Gland, Situated In The Front Part Of The Neck, Is Essential For Controlling The Body's Metabolism Through The Secretion Of Hormones, Mainly Thyroxine (T4) And Triiodothyronine (T3). These Hormones Impact Many Biological Activities Such As Heart Rate, Metabolism, And Energy Levels.

**Hyperthyroidism Is Commonly Caused By:**

**1.** Graves' Disease Is An Autoimmune Condition Characterized By The

Immune System Attacking The Thyroid Gland, Leading To Excessive Hormone Production.

**2.** Toxic Nodular Or Multinodular Goiter Occurs When Nodules Or Tumors On The Thyroid Gland Lead To An Overproduction Of Thyroid Hormones.

**3.** Thyroiditis Is The Inflammation Of The Thyroid Gland That Can Result In A Transient Release Of Stored Hormones, Leading To A Temporary Hyperthyroid Condition.

**4.** Excessive Iodine Consumption, Whether From Food Or Prescription, Can Result In Hyperthyroidism.

**Typical Indications Of Hyperthyroidism Are:**

• Individuals With Hyperthyroidism May Experience Accidental Weight Loss Despite Having An Increased Appetite.

• Increased Heart Rate: Tachycardia And Palpitations Are Frequent Symptoms.

• Excessive Thyroid Hormones Might Cause Heightened Anxiousness And Anxiety.

• Hand And Finger Tremors May Be Observed.

• Heat Intolerance: People With Hyperthyroidism May Struggle To Tolerate High Temperatures.

• Some Folks May Paradoxically Suffer Weariness And Weakness.

• Menstrual Pattern Alterations: Women May Observe Variations In Their Menstrual Cycles.

• Enlarged Thyroid (Goiter): Occasionally, The Thyroid Gland May Grow In Size And Become Noticeable.

Diagnosis Usually Includes Blood Testing To Assess Levels Of Thyroid Hormones (T3 And T4) And Thyroid-Stimulating Hormone (TSH). Imaging Investigations Like Ultrasonography Or Radioactive Iodine Scans Can Be Utilized To Evaluate The Thyroid Gland's Size And Function.

**Possible Treatments For Hyperthyroidism May Comprise:**

• Antithyroid Medications Such As Methimazole Or Propylthiouracil Can Decrease The Synthesis Of Thyroid Hormones.

• Radioactive Iodine Therapy: This Treatment Entails Consuming Radioactive Iodine, Which Specifically Targets And Eliminates Thyroid Cells.

• Thyroidectomy Is The Surgical Procedure Of Removing A Portion Or The Entire Thyroid Gland, Which May Be Advised In Specific Situations.

Hyperthyroidism Management Typically Requires A Multidisciplinary Approach Involving Endocrinologists,

Primary Care Physicians, And Occasionally Surgeons. Consistent Monitoring Is Crucial To Modify Treatment As Necessary And Handle Potential Problems. Individuals With Hyperthyroidism Should Collaborate Closely With Their Healthcare Team To Create A Tailored Treatment Plan That Aligns With Their Unique Condition And Health State.

# Definition and Etiology

Hyperthyroidism Is A Disorder When The Thyroid Gland Is Overactive, Leading To An Excess Production And Release Of Thyroid Hormones Thyroxine (T4) And Triiodothyronine (T3). These Hormones Are Crucial For Controlling Many Metabolic Processes In The Body, Such As Heart Rate, Energy Expenditure, And Temperature.

• **Causes:** Hyperthyroidism Can Result From Various Sources, With The Exact Cause Frequently Dictating The Particular Type Of The Condition. Common Causes Are:

**1. Graves' Disease:** Graves 'disease is An Autoimmune Condition Characterized by the Production of Antibodies That Cause the Thyroid Gland to Release Excessive Hormones. It Is The Primary Cause Of Hyperthyroidism.

**2. Toxic Nodular or Multinodular Goiter:** Nodules Or Lumps May Form On The Thyroid Gland, Resulting In Heightened Hormone Production. This Can Happen In A Solitary Nodule (Toxic Adenoma) Or In Numerous Nodules (Toxic Multinodular Goiter).

**3. Thyroiditis:** Inflammation Of The Thyroid Gland, Typically Triggered By Viral Infections Or Autoimmune Mechanisms, Can Lead To A Transient

Discharge Of Stored Thyroid Hormones. Subtypes Include Of Subacute Thyroiditis, Postpartum Thyroiditis, And Silent Thyroiditis.

**4. Hyperiodism:** Consuming An Excessive Amount Of Iodine From Various Sources Might Cause Hyperthyroidism.

**5. Tumors:** Tumors In The Thyroid Or Pituitary Gland Can Occasionally Cause An Overproduction Of Thyroid-Stimulating Hormone (TSH) Or Thyroid Hormones, Resulting In Hyperthyroidism.

**6. Thyroiditis-Induced Inflammation:** Hashimoto's Thyroiditis, An Autoimmune Illness That Usually Results In Hypothyroidism, Can Sometimes Create A Transient Period Of Hyperthyroidism Due To Inflammation And The Release Of Stored Hormones.

**7. Prescribed Drugs:** Some Drugs, Including Amiodarone For Heart Arrhythmias Or Lithium For Bipolar Disorder, Can Lead To Hyperthyroidism.

• Identifying The Precise Cause Of Hyperthyroidism Is Essential For Selecting The Most Suitable Treatment Method. Medical Practitioners

Frequently Utilize A Blend Of Blood Tests, Imaging Examinations, And Clinical Evaluations To Identify The Root Reason And Customize Treatment Accordingly.

Individuals Showing Signs Of Hyperthyroidism, Like Fast Heart Rate, Weight Loss, And Anxiety, Should Promptly Seek Medical Help. Timely Identification And Management Can Effectively Control The Disease And Avoid Possible Problems.

# Clinical Manifestations and Identification

**Hyperthyroidism Symptoms:** Hyperthyroidism Symptoms Can Range In Intensity And May Encompass:

1. **Weight Loss:** Despite A Heightened Hunger, Individuals May Nevertheless Undergo Inadvertent Weight Loss.

2. **Increased Heart Rate:** Tachycardia And Palpitations Are Frequently Experienced Symptoms.

3. Excessive Thyroid Hormones Might Cause Increased Anxiousness And Anxiety.

4. Hand And Finger Tremors May Be Observed.

5. **Heat Intolerance:** Inability to Tolerate Heat And Excessive Sweating.

6. Paradoxically, Some People May Also Feel Weariness And Weakness.

7. **Muscle Weakness:** Specifically, Weakness In The Upper Arms And Thighs.

8. **Menstrual Pattern Changes**: Women May Observe Anomalies In Their Menstrual Cycles, Like Lighter Or Less Frequent Periods.

9. Insomnia Is Characterized By Difficulty Sleeping.

10. **Heightened Bowel Motions:** Diarrhea And Increased Frequency Of Bowel Motions.
11. **Goiter:** The Thyroid Gland May Appear Swollen And Can Be Felt In The Neck.

Graves 'disease, A Frequent Cause Of Hyperthyroidism, Can Result In Visual Manifestations Such Protruding Eyes (Exophthalmos), Red Or Irritated Eyes, And Alterations In Vision.

## Evaluation:

## 1. Hematological Analysis:

• Thyroid Function Tests (TFTS) Assess Levels Of Thyroid Hormones (T3 And T4) And Thyroid-Stimulating Hormone (TSH). Elevated Levels Of T3

And T4 Are Observed In Hyperthyroidism, With TSH Levels Usually Being Modest.

## 2. Diagnostic Imaging:

• Thyroid Ultrasound Is A Non-Invasive Imaging Technique Used To Evaluate The Size And Structure Of The Thyroid Gland.

• Radioactive Iodine Uptake (RAIU) Scan Is A Test That Detects How Iodine Is Distributed In The Thyroid And Can Indicate Nodules Or Areas With Higher Activity.

## 3. Supplementary Examinations:

• Thyroid Antibody Tests Are Undertaken To Detect Autoimmune Causes By Checking For Antibodies

Such Thyroid-Stimulating Immunoglobulin (TSI) Or Thyroid Peroxidase Antibodies (TPO Antibodies).

• An EKG (Electrocardiogram) Is Used To Evaluate Cardiac Rhythm And Identify Any Irregularities Linked To Hyperthyroidism.

## 4. Clinical Evaluation:

• Perform A Comprehensive Medical History And Physical Examination, Which Includes Evaluating Symptoms and Indicators Such an Enlarged Thyroid Gland or Eye Abnormalities (With Graves 'disease).

## 5. Fine-Needle Aspiration (FNA):

• If Nodules Are Found, A Fine-Needle Aspiration May Be Done To Exclude Thyroid Cancer.

The Treatment Plan For Hyperthyroidism Is Determined By Identifying The Specific Underlying Cause, Such As Graves' Disease, Toxic Nodular Goiter, Or Another Ailment. Management Of Thyroid Overactivity Typically Includes A Mix Of Drugs, Radioactive Iodine Therapy, Or Surgery. Consistent Monitoring Is Essential To Maintain Optimal Thyroid Hormone Levels And Address Any Possible Problems. People With Signs Of Hyperthyroidism Should Promptly Seek Medical Attention For A

# Comprehensive Evaluation And Diagnosis.

# CHAPTER TWO
## Consequences of Unmanaged Hyperthyroidism

Unmanaged Hyperthyroidism Can Result In Diverse Problems, Impacting Several Organ Systems In The Body. It Is Essential To Promptly Seek Medical Care And Adhere To A Treatment Regimen To Effectively Control Hyperthyroidism And Avoid Possible Consequences. Complications Of Untreated Hyperthyroidism Include:

## 1. Cardiovascular Issues:

• Arrhythmias Can Occur Due To Prolonged High Levels Of Thyroid Hormones, Causing Irregular Heartbeats.

Untreated Hyperthyroidism Can Lead To Heart Failure In Severe Cases Due To The Strain It Puts On The Heart.

**2. Concerns Related To Bone Health:** Untreated Hyperthyroidism Can Speed Up Bone Metabolism, Resulting In Decreased Bone Density (Osteoporosis) And A Higher Likelihood Of Fractures.

**3. Thyroid Storm:** Untreated Hyperthyroidism Can Sometimes Result In A Life-Threatening Disease Called Thyroid Storm, Which Is Marked By Significant Increases In Heart Rate, Body Temperature, And Blood Pressure.

**4. Ocular Complications In Graves' Disease:** Graves' Illness, A Frequent Source Of Hyperthyroidism, Can Result In Eye Issues Include Protruding Eyes (Exophthalmos), Double Vision, And Alterations In Vision. Vision Loss May Occur In Severe Cases.

**5. Mental and Brain-Related Problems:** Untreated Hyperthyroidism Can Lead To Heightened Anxiety, Nervousness, And Mood Disruptions. Sometimes, It Might Result In Cognitive Impairments Such As Problems With Focus And Recollection.

## 6. Gastrointestinal Problems:

• Increased Bowel Motions And Diarrhea Are Prevalent Signs Of Hyperthyroidism. Untreated Hyperthyroidism Can Lead To Gastrointestinal Problems And Weight Loss.

## 7. Reproductive Problems:

Untreated Hyperthyroidism In Women Can Lead To Irregular Menstrual Periods And Reproductive Issues. Pregnant Women With Uncontrolled Hyperthyroidism Face A Higher Likelihood Of Problems Such As Preterm Birth And Low Birth Weight.

**8.    Dermatological   And   Pilose Changes:** Hyperthyroidism Can Lead To Alterations In The Skin, Such As Thinning And Heightened Fragility. Hair Might Become Fragile And Susceptible To Breaking.

## 9. Muscle Weakness and Atrophy:

• Chronic Hyperthyroidism Can Result In Muscular Atrophy And Debility, Impacting Overall Physical Prowess And Functionality.

## 10.   Heightened   Susceptibility   To Infections:

**Infections:** The Immune System May Be Weakened, Making The Individual More Prone To Infections.

The Severity And Likelihood Of Problems In Hyperthyroidism Can

Differ Among Individuals And Are Influenced By Factors Like The Underlying Etiology, Duration Of The Condition, And Individual Health Characteristics. Timely Identification And Proper Treatment Can Greatly Decrease The Likelihood Of Complications Linked To Hyperthyroidism. Those With Signs Of Hyperthyroidism Should Get A Comprehensive Examination And Treatment Plan From A Healthcare Provider.

# The Impact of Diet on Thyroid Function

Nutrition Is Essential For Maintaining Optimal Thyroid Function, As Specific Nutrients Are Vital For Producing And Controlling Thyroid Hormones. Diet Alone Cannot Treat Thyroid Diseases, But It Can Help Maintain A Healthy Thyroid And Manage Symptoms. Here Are Several Ways Nutrition Impacts Thyroid Function:

## 1. Iodine:

• Iodine Plays A Crucial Role In The Production Of Thyroid Hormones (T3 And T4). Optimal Iodine Consumption Is Crucial For Maintaining Thyroid Health. Inadequate Iodine Can Cause Hypothyroidism, Whereas Much

Iodine Might Worsen Hyperthyroidism.

## 2. Selenium

- Selenium Is A Vital Mineral That Is A Component Of Enzymes Responsible For Converting Inactive T4 To Active T3 Thyroid Hormone. Selenium Aids In Safeguarding The Thyroid Gland Against Oxidative Harm.

## 3. Zinc:

- Zinc Is A Crucial Mineral For Thyroid Function Because It Plays A Role In The Production Of Thyroid Hormones. Zinc Insufficiency Can Affect Thyroid Function.

## 4. Iron:

• Iron Is Essential For The Optimal Functioning Of Thyroid Peroxidase, An Enzyme Crucial For The Synthesis Of Thyroid Hormones. Iron Deficiency Can Impact The Synthesis Of Thyroid Hormones.

## 5. Vitamin D:

• Vitamin D Is Involved In The Function Of Thyroid Hormone Receptors, And A Lack Of It Has Been Associated With Autoimmune Thyroid Disorders. Sufficient Vitamin D Levels Are Crucial For General Well-Being And Can Have A Beneficial Impact On Thyroid Function.

## 6. Tyrosine Is An Amino Acid.

• Tyrosine Is An Amino Acid That Reacts With Iodine To Create Thyroid Hormones. A Protein-Rich Diet Supplies Essential Components, Such As Tyrosine, Needed For The Production Of Thyroid Hormones.

## 7. Cruciferous Vegetables:

• Cruciferous Plants Like Broccoli, Cabbage, And Kale Have Chemicals That Can Disrupt Thyroid Function In Excessive Quantities, But Are Often Safe For Those With Normal Thyroid Function When Consumed In Moderate Amounts. Cooking Can Mitigate Potential Adverse Effects.

## 8. Avoiding Goitrogenic Foods:

• Certain Foods, Called Goitrogens, Can Disrupt Iodine Absorption And Thyroid Activity. These Consist Of Specific Uncooked Cruciferous Veggies, Soy, And Some Fruits. Cooking Can Diminish The Goitrogenic Impact.

## 9. Preventing Excessive Iodine Consumption:

• Consuming Too Much Iodine, Whether From Food Or Supplements, Can Lead To Thyroid Problems. This Is Especially Important For Persons With Preexisting Thyroid Disorders.

• Individual Responses To Dietary Modifications Might Vary, And What

Works For One Person May Not Be Good For Another. Dietary Recommendations May Vary Based On The Exact Type Of Thyroid Illness (Hypothyroidism, Hyperthyroidism, Autoimmune Thyroid Diseases) And Their Root Causes.

If You Have Worries About Your Thyroid Function Or Have Been Diagnosed With A Thyroid Condition, It Is Essential To Seek Advice From A Healthcare Practitioner Or A Certified Dietitian. They Can Offer Tailored Guidance According To Your Individual Health Requirements And Factors To Consider. Make Dietary Changes In Consultation With Your

Healthcare Provider To Ensure They Align With Your Treatment Plan.

# CHAPTER THREE
## Hyperthyroidism Diet: Recommended Foods

Individuals With Hyperthyroidism Require A Diet That Is Well-Balanced And Rich In Nutrients. Dietary Changes Cannot Cure Hyperthyroidism But Can Assist In Symptom Management And Promote Overall Health. Here Are Some Foods That May Be Good In A Diet Suitable For Hyperthyroidism:

## 1. Low-Fat Proteins:

• Include Lean Protein Sources Including Poultry, Fish, Tofu, Lentils, And Low-Fat Dairy In Your Diet. Protein Is Crucial For Preserving

Muscle Mass, Particularly When Focusing On Weight Loss.

## 2. Whole Grains:

• Select Whole Grains Such As Brown Rice, Quinoa, Whole Wheat, And Oats. This Food Source Offers Intricate Carbs And Fiber, Which Help Maintain Consistent Energy Levels.

## 3. Monounsaturated and Polyunsaturated Fats:

• Incorporate Sources Of Healthy Fats Including Avocados, Nuts, Seeds, And Olive Oil. These Fats Are Crucial For General Well-Being And Can Help Increase Calorie Consumption In Those Experiencing Weight Loss Due To Hyperthyroidism.

## 4. Produce:

• Strive To Include A Diverse Selection Of Vibrant Fruits And Vegetables In Your Diet, As They Are Abundant In Vitamins, Minerals, And Antioxidants. These Can Promote General Well-Being And Supply Vital Nutrients.

## 5. Foods Low in Iodine:

• Individuals With Hyperthyroidism Caused By Iodine Sensitivity Should Restrict Their Intake Of Iodine-Rich Foods Including Seaweed, Iodized Salt, And Some Types Of Seafood. Choose Low-Iodine Options.

## 6. Dairy or Dairy Substitutes:

• Include Dairy Products Or Fortified Dairy Alternatives To Enhance Bone

Health With Calcium And Vitamin D. Hyperthyroidism Can Impact Bone Density, Hence It Is Crucial To Ensure Sufficient Calcium Intake.

## 7. Hydrating Drinks:

• Maintain Good Hydration By Consuming Water, Herbal Teas, And Other Non-Caffeinated Drinks. Dehydration Can Lead To Symptoms Such As Weariness.

## 8. Cruciferous Vegetables That Have Been Prepared By Cooking.

• Cooking Cruciferous Vegetables Can Decrease Their Goitrogenic Impact By Breaking Down The Chemicals That May Disrupt Thyroid Function. Incorporate Moderate Quantities Of

Cooked Broccoli, Cauliflower, Cabbage, And Brussels Sprouts.

## 9. Consistent, Modest Portions:

• Consume Smaller, More Frequent Meals Over The Day To Maintain Energy Levels And Manage Potential Weight Changes.

## 10. Avoid Excessive Use Of Stimulants.

• Avoid Or Cut Down On Caffeine And Nicotine, As These Might Worsen Symptoms Such As Anxiety And Insomnia.

## 11. Supplements Of Vitamins And Minerals:

• Your Healthcare Professional May Suggest Specific Vitamin Or Mineral Supplements Like Selenium, Zinc, Or B Vitamins Based On Your Individual Needs And Inadequacies.

Individual Responses To Dietary Modifications Can Vary, Therefore It Is Crucial To Collaborate Closely With Your Healthcare Team, Particularly A Licensed Dietitian Or Nutritionist. They Offer Tailored Advice According To Your Individual Health Requirements, Track Nutritional Status, And Guarantee Dietary Adjustments Are In Line With Your Treatment Plan. Regularly Meeting

With Your Healthcare Physician Is
Essential To Evaluate Thyroid
Hormone Levels And Modify
Treatment If Necessary.

## Avoid These Foods If You Have Hyperthyroidism

There Is No Universal Dietary Plan For
Hyperthyroidism, Although It Is
Recommended To Restrict Or Avoid
Particular Foods Based On Individual
Sensitivities And The Root Cause Of
The Disorder. Here Are Some General
Tips On Foods To Restrict Or Avoid
When Dealing With Hyperthyroidism:

**1. Foods Rich in Iodine:**

• Excessive Iodine Consumption Might
Worsen Hyperthyroidism. Avoid

Consuming Foods High In Iodine, Such As Iodized Salt, Seaweed, Seafood, And Specific Dairy Products.

## 2. Raw Cruciferous Vegetables:

• Cruciferous Vegetables Such As Broccoli, Cauliflower, Cabbage, And Brussels Sprouts Contain Goitrogens That Can Disrupt Thyroid Function. Cooking These Vegetables Can Decrease Their Goitrogenic Effects.

## 3. Soy and Soy Products:

Soy Includes Is flavones That Can Disrupt The Absorption Of Thyroid Hormones. It Is Recommended To Restrict The Consumption Of Soy-Based Goods.

## 4. Caffeinated Drinks:

• Excessive Consumption Of Caffeine Can Lead To Symptoms Such As Elevated Heart Rate And Heightened Anxiety. Avoid Or Restrict Consumption Of Caffeinated Beverages Such As Coffee, Tea, And Energy Drinks.

## 5. Processed and Sugary Foods:

• Highly Processed Diets And Those Rich In Refined Sugars Can Lead To Inflammation And Disturb Hormonal Equilibrium. Choose Full, Unprocessed Meals And Restrict Added Sugars.

**6. Alcohol:** Excessive Alcohol Intake Can Disrupt Thyroid Function And Harm The Liver, Which Plays A Role In

Thyroid Hormone Processing. Restrict Alcohol Consumption.

## 7. High-Fat and Deep-Fried Foods:

• Reduce Consumption Of High-Fat And Fried Foods To Minimize Inflammation And Weight Gain, Which Are Potential Issues In Hyperthyroidism.

## 8. High Fiber Intake:

• Excessive Fiber Intake Can Hinder The Absorption Of Thyroid Medicines, Despite Its Usual Benefits For Digestive Health. Consume A Well-Rounded Amount Of Fiber Without Overdoing Supplements.

## 9. Overabundance Of Vitamin And Mineral Supplements:

• Consuming High Doses Of Specific Vitamins And Minerals Like Iodine Or Selenium Without Medical Oversight Might Lead To Adverse Consequences. Seek Advice From Your Healthcare Physician Prior To Consuming Supplements.

## 10. Dairy (Occasionally):

• Dairy Products Can Cause Gastrointestinal Problems In People With Lactose Intolerance Or Sensitivity. Select Lactose-Free Options If Needed.

Dietary Recommendations May Differ Depending On Individual Health

Circumstances, The Precise Cause Of Hyperthyroidism, And The Presence Of Other Medical Disorders. Prior To Making Substantial Alterations To Your Dietary Habits, Particularly While Managing A Medical Condition Such As Hyperthyroidism, It Is Essential To Seek Advice From Your Healthcare Provider Or A Trained Dietitian. They Can Offer Tailored Guidance, Considering Your Individual Health Requirements And Factors. Consistent Check-Ins With Your Healthcare Team Are Crucial For Monitoring Thyroid Hormone Levels And Making Therapy Adjustments As Necessary.

# CHAPTER FOUR

## Meal Planning For Hyperthyroidism

Planning Meals For Hyperthyroidism Requires Selecting Foods That Are Rich In Nutrients To Promote General Well-Being And Address Symptoms Linked To An Overactive Thyroid. Below Is An Example Meal Plan That Offers A Range Of Foods Rich In Essential Nutrients For Those With Hyperthyroidism.

**First Meal of the Day:**

**1. Quinoa Breakfast Bowl:**

- Cooked Quinoa Sliced Bananas
- Chopped Nuts Like Walnuts Or Almonds, Greek Yogurt Or A Dairy Free Option, And A

Drizzle Of Honey Or Maple Syrup.

- Sprinkle Chia Seeds for Additional Fiber, If Desired.

## 2. Mid-Morning Snack:

- 2. Apple and Nut Butter:
- Slices Of Apple
- Almond, Peanut, Or Sunflower Seed Butter

## 3. Lunch: Grilled Chicken Salad

- Grilled Chicken Breast
- Assorted Greens (Spinach, Kale, Arugula)
- Cherry Tomatoes
- Sliced Cucumber
- Quinoa or Brown Rice

- Dressing Made Of Olive Oil And Lemon

**4. Afternoon Snack**: Greek Yogurt Parfait:

- Greek Yogurt
- Assorted Berries (Blueberries, Strawberries)
- Granola (Low-Sugar And Whole Grain) Optional: A Dash Of Flaxseeds Or Pumpkin Seeds For Extra Nutrients

**Dinner:** Baked Salmon With Sweet Potato And Asparagus At 5 O'clock.

- Baked Salmon Fillet

- Roasted Sweet Potato Wedges

- Steamed Asparagus

- Drizzle With Olive Oil And Sprinkle With Herbs Such As Rosemary Or Thyme

**6. Evening Snack (Optional):** Hummus with Vegetables:

- Carrot and Cucumber Sticks

- Hummus For Dipping

**Hydration:**

- Stay Well-Hydrated By Drinking Ample Water throughout the Day.

- Consider Herbal Teas Like Chamomile Or Peppermint As Suitable Options.

**Factors to Take Into Account:**

• Use Caution With Iodine Consumption, Particularly If Hyperthyroidism Is Linked To Iodine Sensitivity. Restrict The Consumption Of Iodized Salt And High-Iodine Foods Such As Seaweed And Specific Types Of Seafood.

• Soy Awareness: Individuals With Hyperthyroidism Should Restrict Soy Products Because Of Their Possible Effect On Thyroid Function.

• Consistent, Nutritious Meals: Strive For Consistent Meals And Snacks To Sustain Energy Levels And Avoid Unintended Weight Loss.

This Meal Plan Offers A Diverse Range Of Nutrients Such As Protein, Healthy Fats, Fiber, Vitamins, And Minerals. Customizing Your Meal Plan Is Crucial To Accommodate Personal Tastes, Dietary Limitations, And Special Health Requirements. Seeking Guidance From A Certified Dietitian Or Nutritionist Can Assist In Developing A Customized Food Plan That Meets Your Specific Needs And Promotes Your Overall Health. Regularly Scheduled Appointments With Your Healthcare Provider Are Essential For Monitoring Thyroid Hormone Levels And Making Necessary Adjustments To Your Treatment Plan.

## Supplements for Thyroid Support

Individuals With Thyroid Issues May Opt For Supplements To Enhance Thyroid Function In Addition To Maintaining A Balanced Diet Rich In Key Nutrients. It Is Important To Emphasize That The Consumption Of Supplements Should Be Supervised By A Healthcare Professional, As An Excessive Amount Of Specific Nutrients Can Lead To Negative Consequences. Here Are Some Substances That Could Be Used To Help The Thyroid:

• Iodine Is An Essential Element In Thyroid Hormones. Excessive Iodine Consumption Can Exacerbate Several Thyroid Problems, Particularly In

Persons With Iodine Sensitivity. It Is Crucial To Obtain Iodine From Food Sources And Seek Advice From A Healthcare Professional If Considering Supplementation.

• Selenium Is Necessary For The Conversion Of The Dormant Thyroid Hormone T4 To The Active Thyroid Hormone T3. Research Indicates That Selenium Supplementation May Be Advantageous For Persons With Autoimmune Thyroid Diseases Such As Hashimoto's Thyroiditis Or Graves' Disease. Excessive Selenium Use Might Be Detrimental, Therefore, It Is Advisable To Seek Guidance From A Healthcare Practitioner Prior To Using Supplements.

• Zinc Is Involved In The Synthesis Of Thyroid Hormones. Sufficient Zinc Levels Are Crucial For Optimal Thyroid Function. Zinc Supplementation Is Typically Advised For Individuals With A Verified Deficit.

• Vitamin D Plays A Role In The Action Of Thyroid Hormone Receptors. Vitamin D Deficiency Is Associated With Autoimmune Thyroid Disorders. If Your Vitamin D Levels Are Low, Your Healthcare Professional May Suggest Supplementation.

• Vitamin B Complex, Which Includes B12 And Folate, Is Involved In Energy Metabolism And May Help In Maintaining Thyroid Function. People With Deficits May Find B-Complex

Vitamins Helpful, But It Is Crucial To Identify And Address Particular Deficiencies Through Testing.

• Iron Is Essential For The Normal Functioning Of Thyroid Peroxidase, An Enzyme That Plays A Role In Synthesizing Thyroid Hormones. Iron Insufficiency Can Affect Thyroid Function, And Supplementation May Be Advised In Cases Of Deficiency.

• Omega-3 Fatty Acids, Present In Fish Oil Supplements, May Possess Anti-Inflammatory Properties That Could Be Advantageous For Patients With Autoimmune Thyroid Problems. It Is Crucial To Acquire Omega-3s From Food Sources And To Contemplate

Supplementation With Medical Oversight.

Prior To Using Any Supplements, It Is Essential To Seek Advice From A Healthcare Specialist, Ideally One Specializing In Endocrinology Or Thyroid Conditions. They Can Evaluate Your Specific Health Requirements, Perform Relevant Tests To Pinpoint Inadequacies, And Establish The Most Appropriate Vitamins And Dosages For You. Taking Supplements Without Sufficient Counsel Might Cause Imbalances And Significant Health Hazards. Consistent Monitoring And Follow-Ups With Your Healthcare Team Are Crucial To Verify That Supplements Are In Line With Your

Entire Treatment Plan And Health Objectives.

# CHAPTER FIVE
## Techniques for Retaining Nutrients in Cooking

Cooking Methods Can Greatly Affect The Nutritional Value Of Meals. Specific Procedures Aid In Maintaining The Vitamins, Minerals, And Other Useful Substances Found In The Foods. Here Are Cooking Techniques That Often Preserve Nutrients:

• Steaming Is A Delicate Cooking Technique That Involves Exposing Food To Low Levels Of Heat And Water. It Aids In Maintaining The Color, Texture, And Nutrient Composition Of Vegetables, Fish, And Other Food Items.

• Microwaving Is A Rapid And Effective Cooking Technique That Can Preserve More Nutrients Than Certain Other Ways. It Necessitates Less Water Usage And Shorter Cooking Durations.

• Sautéing Is The Process Of Rapidly Frying Food In A Small Quantity Of Oil On Medium Heat. This Approach Preserves The Color And Nutrition Of Veggies While Enhancing Flavor.

• Blanching Is The Process Of Momentarily Submerging Vegetables In Hot Water And Then Quickly Cooling Them. This Approach Aids In Maintaining The Color, Texture, And Nutritional Content Of Vegetables.

• Grilling And Broiling Involve Using Direct Heat From Either Above (Broiling) Or Below (Grilling) To Rapidly Cook Food. These Techniques Can Preserve Nutrients While Imparting A Smokey Taste.

• Baking And Roasting Involve Subjecting Food To Dry Heat In An Oven. These Techniques Can Preserve Nutrients Effectively, Particularly By Employing Lower Temperatures And Shorter Cooking Durations.

• Slow Cooking Is The Process Of Boiling Food At Low Temperatures Over A Long Period Of Time. Although It May Result In Nutrient Loss, This Method Is Convenient For Maintaining

The Tastes And Suppleness Of Ingredients.

• Pressure Cooking Utilizes Steam And High Pressure To Rapidly Cook Food. It Can Help Preserve More Nutrients Than Regular Boiling By Reducing The Cooking Time.

• Consuming Fruits, Vegetables, And Certain Proteins Raw Or Mildly Cooked Can Optimize Nutritional Absorption. It Is Important To Take Into Account Individual Tastes And Digestive Tolerance.

• Utilize Cooking Water From Boiling Or Steaming Vegetables In Other Recipes To Retain Water-Soluble

Nutrients That May Dissolve Into The Water.

• Overcooking, Excessive Heat, And Lengthy Cooking Durations Can Result In Nutritional Loss. Furthermore, Selecting Fresh, High-Quality Ingredients And Appropriate Storage Methods Can Help Maintain Nutrient Levels.

Although Various Cooking Techniques Can Aid In Retaining Nutrients, The Overall Balance And Diversity Of Foods In Your Diet Are Crucial For Fulfilling Nutritional Requirements. Individual Nutrient Needs Can Vary Depending On Factors Like Age, Gender, Health Condition, And Lifestyle. Seeking Guidance From A

Certified Dietitian Or Nutritionist Can Offer Tailored Recommendations According To Your Individual Dietary Requirements And Choices.

## Monitoring and Modifying Your Diet

Monitoring And Modifying Your Food Can Be A Beneficial Strategy To Ensure You Are Fulfilling Your Nutritional Requirements, Particularly When Dealing With Diseases Such As Hyperthyroidism. Here Are Steps To Efficiently Monitor And Modify Your Diet:

• Maintain A Food Journal By Documenting All Food And Beverages Consumed During The Day. Provide Specifics Like Serving Sizes,

Preparation Techniques, And Any Symptoms Or Fluctuations In Energy Levels You See.

• Utilize A Nutrition App To Monitor Your Daily Food Consumption. Several Applications Offer Databases Of Food Items With Nutritional Data, Facilitating The Tracking Of Nutrient Consumption.

• Monitor Essential Nutrients Crucial For Thyroid Function, Including Iodine, Selenium, Zinc, And Vitamins D And B12. Monitor Your Consumption To Make Sure You Are Reaching The Required Levels.

• Monitor Your Thyroid Hormone Levels Regularly By Collaborating

With Your Healthcare Professional To Set Up A Testing Regimen. This Might Aid In Detecting Any Variations That May Necessitate Modifications To Your Treatment Plan Or Eating Strategy.

• Seek Advice From A Registered Dietitian: A Registered Dietitian Specializing In Thyroid Health Can Offer Tailored Recommendations. They Can Assist You In Comprehending Your Nutritional Requirements, Provide Dietary Suggestions, And Deal With Any Issues Or Obstacles You May Face.

• Monitor Your Body's Reactions To Various Foods And Modify Your Diet Accordingly Based On Symptoms. If You Have Heightened Anxiety Or

Palpitations After Ingesting Specific Foods Or Drinks, You Should Adjust Your Consumption.

• Implement Dietary Modifications Gradually. This Enables Your Body To Adjust And Enhances Your Ability To Recognize The Impacts Of Particular Alterations.

• Maintain Proper Fluids For Optimal Health. Make Careful To Stay Adequately Hydrated During The Day, As Dehydration Can Lead To Weariness And Other Symptoms.

• Consider The Timing Of Your Meals And Be Mindful Of When You Consume Food. Individuals With Hyperthyroidism May Find It Helpful

To Consume Smaller, More Frequent Meals To Help Control Symptoms Like Weight Loss And Heightened Metabolism.

• Assess Your Energy Levels And Overall Well-Being. If You Have Ongoing Exhaustion Or Fluctuations In Energy, Seek Advice From Your Healthcare Professional To Investigate Possible Reasons.

• Incorporate Regular Exercise To Promote Overall Health And Potentially Regulate Weight Changes Linked To Hyperthyroidism. Seek Advice From Your Healthcare Practitioner Before Initiating A New Workout Routine.

Keep In Mind That Each Individual's Physique Is Distinct, And A Method That Is Effective For One Person May Not Be Effective For Another. It Is Essential To Have Clear Communication With Your Healthcare Providers, Such As Your Endocrinologist And Dietitian, To Make Sure That Your Diet Is Suitable For Your Individual Health Requirements And Treatment Regimen. Consistent Monitoring And Modifications To Your Diet And Therapy Are Crucial Aspects Of Effectively Treating Hyperthyroidism.

# Conclusion

Managing Hyperthyroidism Requires A Holistic Approach That Encompasses Medical Therapy, Lifestyle Adjustments, And Dietary Concerns. Individuals Diagnosed With Hyperthyroidism Must Comprehend The Condition, Its Symptoms, And Potential Complications.

It Is Essential To Follow A Well-Rounded Diet That Promotes General Health And Meets Individual Nutritional Requirements. This May Require Including Nutrient-Rich Meals Like Lean Proteins, Whole Grains, Fruits, And Vegetables, While Considering Specific Dietary

Limitations Linked To Hyperthyroidism.

Monitoring Your Nutrition, Maintaining Hydration, And Adapting Eating Habits According To Symptoms And Thyroid Hormone Levels Are Crucial Tactics. Seeking Advice From Healthcare Experts Such As Endocrinologists And Qualified Dietitians Can Offer Tailored Recommendations And Guarantee That Dietary Modifications Are In Harmony With Your Comprehensive Treatment Strategy.

Lifestyle Variables Including Consistent Physical Activity, Effective Stress Control, And Adequate Sleep

Contribute To Maintaining Thyroid Health And Overall Wellness.

Hyperthyroidism Can Be Effectively Managed With Appropriate Medical Treatment And Lifestyle Changes. Consistent Communication With Your Healthcare Team, Following Prescribed Treatments, And Taking A Proactive Approach To Your Food And Lifestyle Can Lead To Improved Results And A Higher Quality Of Life. If You Have Or Think You Have Hyperthyroidism, Promptly Seek Medical Help For A Comprehensive Evaluation And Tailored Treatment Plan.

**THE END**